SECOND CHANCE AT 75

SECOND CHANCE AT 75

ELECTIVE BUT URGENT CABG AND CAROTID ENDARTERECTOMY

JAWAD HASNAIN MD, MBA, FACC

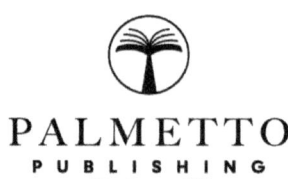

PALMETTO
PUBLISHING
Charleston, SC
www.PalmettoPublishing.com

Copyright © 2024 by Jawad Hasnain

All rights reserved

No portion of this book may be reproduced, stored in a retrieval system, or transmitted in any form by any means—electronic, mechanical, photocopy, recording, or other—except for brief quotations in printed reviews, without prior permission of the author.

Hardcover ISBN: 979-8-8229-7147-9
Paperback ISBN: 979-8-8229-5493-9
eBook ISBN: 979-8-8229-5494-6

This book is dedicated to my parents, Sarfraz Sibtain and Mohammed Sibtain, who instilled in me a lifelong passion for acquiring knowledge, being truthful, and helping others.

> Hein Loeg wohi jahan mein achaiy
> Aate hein jo kaam duusaroen kaiy.
>
> Earn nobility through serving humanity.
>
> —Allama Iqbal

I am also extremely grateful for the excellent medical care I received at John Hopkins Medicine in the Department of Cardiovascular Surgery (Dr. Hamza Aziz) and the Department of Vascular Surgery (Dr. James Black III) and from my primary care physician (Dr. Saba Sheikh).

I am indebted to the whole peri-operative team. Thanks a lot for giving me a second chance.

We bestowed all the knowledge upon Muhammad. He will teach you knowledge and wisdom and purify you.

—Al-Quran 62:3

Anaa Madintul Ilm e wa Ali un Babohah.

—Holy Prophet's Hadith

I (Muhammad) am the city of knowledge, and Ali is the gateway.

Bismillah ar-Rahman ar-Raheem.
I start with the name of Allah, who is most merciful and most compassionate.

Hadisa jo ke abhi parda e aflak mein hai
Aks uska marey aaina e idrak mein hai
Ilm key haad se parey banda e momin keliyae
Lazat e shoaq be hai nemat e deedar be hai.

Knowledge is the key that opens the doors of perception and discovery of new avenues and ideas.

—Allama Iqbal

Author's Note

Cardiovascular disease and Cerebrovascular disease (Stroke) are the leading causes of morbidity, mortality, and disability with increasing incidence. Heart disease costs the United States about 219 Billion dollars annually. This total amount includes the cost of healthcare services, medications, and premature deaths. Cardiovascular disease costs will exceed One Trillion Dollars by 2035.

The importance of prevention and timely and effective treatment cannot be overemphasized. In this book I describe my experience with these scourges. I have tried to explain these diseases, treatment options, and strategies to prevent and minimize the socioeconomic impact of these diseases. I hope that this educational approach will benefit readers.

CONTENTS

Prologue	xiii
Atherosclerotic Cardiovascular Disease (ASCVD)	1
Cerebrovascular Accidents (CVAs): Strokes and Transient Ischemic Attacks (TIAs)	18
Interventional Therapy	37
Metabolic Syndrome	49
Glossary	61
Medical Terminology	67
Acknowledgments	69
About the Author	71

PROLOGUE

I have been blessed with health all my life. I have pursued a heathy lifestyle comprising proper nutrition, exercise, adequate sleep, and spiritual peace. I have a very satisfying medical career. My passion and profession are aligned. I have been blessed with loving family and friends.

A few weeks after my seventy-fifth birthday, my life changed. It all started with partial numbness of the right side of my body for a few weeks prior. This prompted a medical workup after consultation with my primary care physician. Over the next week and a half, I underwent medical investigations, tests, and consultation with various medical professionals. This workup led to elective (although urgent) left carotid endarterectomy followed the next morning by triple coronary artery bypass surgery to prevent potential but imminent life-threatening complications, including stroke, heart attack, and death. Both surgeries were successful, and I suffered no complications.

This all transpired despite no signs and symptoms and no functional limitations. It happened to me in spite of my being healthy and active throughout my life.

ATHEROSCLEROTIC CARDIOVASCULAR DISEASE (ASCVD)

Conditions related to atherosclerotic cardiovascular disease (ASCVD) remain the leading cause of morbidity and mortality globally.

ASCVD can present as coronary artery disease (CAD), cerebrovascular disease (CVA), transient ischemic attack (TIA), peripheral artery disease (PAD), and abdominal aneurysms, as well as renal artery stenosis.

ASCVD is caused by plaque buildup in arterial walls and refers to conditions that include the following:
- Coronary artery disease (CAD) such as myocardial infarction, angina, and coronary artery stenosis
- Cerebrovascular disease, such as a transient ischemic attack, ischemic stroke, and carotid artery stenosis
- Peripheral artery disease, such as claudication
- Aortic atherosclerotic disease, such as abdominal aortic aneurysm and descending thoracic aneurysm

Angina pain from a clogged artery is typically felt during exertion, and it usually goes away with rest. Other symptoms may include the following:

- Dizziness
- Feeling like your heart is racing
- Nausea or indigestion
- Shortness of breath
- Sweating

Prevalence
The prevalence of heart disease has decreased over the last decade.
- The age-adjusted prevalence of heart disease in men decreased from 8.3 percent in 2009 to 7 percent in 2019.
- The age-adjusted prevalence of heart disease in women decreased from 4.6 percent in 2009 to 4.2 percent in 2019.
- The prevalence of atherosclerotic cardiovascular disease among adults in the US is 18.3 million (8.0 percent). Last year, 690,524 adults had an acute coronary syndrome event, and over six million are at very high risk.

By the age of forty, about half of us have cholesterol deposits in our arteries, After forty-five, men may have a lot of plaque buildup. Signs of atherosclerosis in women are likely to appear after age fifty-five.

Clogged arteries are caused by a buildup of plaque in arteries. Plaque is usually made up of a few substances, including minerals like calcium, or fats and cholesterol. High cholesterol levels can lead to this buildup of plaque.

In some cases, high cholesterol is genetic, but it is mostly linked to diet and lifestyle choices, including level of exercise, cigarette smoking, and obesity. Eating a diet high in saturated fats, trans fats, and triglycerides is linked to an increased risk of atherosclerosis.

What Is Cholesterol?

Cholesterol is a waxy, fat-like substance that circulates in the blood and is found in the cells of your body. It helps your body build cell membranes, vitamin D, and hormones. However, too much cholesterol can lead to heart health problems. Low-density lipoprotein (LDL) is known as the "bad" cholesterol because it contributes to heart disease by adding to fatty buildup in the arteries. This fatty buildup leads to a narrowing of the arteries and increases the risk of heart attack and stroke. High-density lipoprotein (HDL) is known as the "good" cholesterol because it helps remove some LDL cholesterol from the arteries, which may protect against heart attack and stroke.

Low- and very low-carb diets do seem to offer greater benefits for appetite control, reducing triglycerides, and decreasing the need for medication in people with type 2 diabetes. Studies showed mixed results on LDL (bad) cholesterol levels, with some demonstrating an increase.

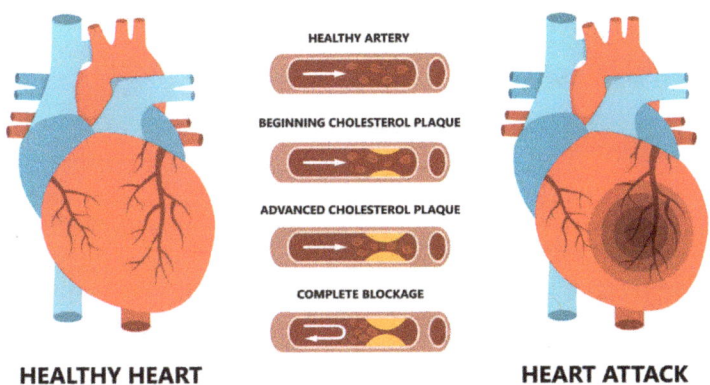

Heart Attack and Stages of Atherosclerosis

Management of High Cholesterol

There is no easy way to unclog an artery once plaque has built up. However, dietary choices, exercise, and avoiding smoking can improve cardiovascular health and stop blockages from worsening. In some cases, medication or surgery may be necessary.

Consider treatment with a moderate- to high-intensity statin. People with an ASCVD risk greater than or equal to 15 percent over ten years should initiate or continue moderate- to high-intensity statin. People with diabetes, aged forty to seventy-five, with ASCVD risk greater than or equal to 7.5 percent over ten years should initiate or continue moderate-intensity statin. Consider use of a high-intensity statin.

The use of statins in diabetic patients can lower the incidence of coronary artery disease or stroke by 24 percent and risk of death by 16 percent. The statins in older patients can increase the risk of side effects, such as muscle pains, liver problems, and increased risk of diabetes in patients with atherosclerotic heart disease; statins offer maximum benefit. The indications for heart disease prevention are still being investigated.

Patients with Atherosclerosis

At present, lowering LDL to less than 100mg/dL is recommended. Use of statins to lower LDL levels below 100mg/dL is beneficial in patients with CHD. Once the diagnosis of acute coronary or cerebrovascular disease is established, statin therapy should be initiated.

The keto diet may affect cholesterol levels, but more research needs to be done before we will know how much and under what circumstances. Cholesterol levels are linked to heart disease risk, so it's important to discuss this diet with your health-care provider before trying it, especially if you have other risk factors. The keto diet differs from other low-carb diets in that it is much more strict in the number of macronutrients allowed. (Macronutrients are carbohydrates, fats, and protein.) These provide calories and energy and make up the greatest amount of nutrients people consume. The keto diet typically limits total carbohydrate intake to only about 5 to 10 percent of your total daily calories, or about twenty to fifty grams a day. The typical fat intake on a keto diet is around 70 to 80 percent of your total daily calories, with 10 to 20 percent of your daily calories coming from protein.

Regular exercise isn't just for those who are looking to prevent heart problems. It can help people whose heart muscle is already damaged. Although exercise can't clear existing plaque from clogged arteries, it can help prevent further accumulation.

Exercise has many positive effects on vascular health:
- Delivers more oxygenated blood throughout the body to keep tissues and organs healthy
- Improves metabolism, which helps control blood glucose, burn fats, and maintain or decrease body weight
- Increases production of nitric oxide, which relaxes the inner muscles of your blood vessels
- Prompts the body to make more capillaries in your muscles, giving muscles more oxygen and increasing muscle efficiency
- Increases mitochondria, small structures inside cells that create energy
- Reduces inflammation throughout the body
- Widens arteries and makes them more flexible, decreasing resistance and blood pressure

With healthy arteries, you have a lower risk of high blood pressure, high cholesterol, and heart failure. This lowers the chances of cardiovascular events such as cardiac death, stroke, and heart attack.

When beginning a new exercise program, talk to your physician (PCP), your cardiologist, an exercise physiologist, or a physical therapist. They can advise you on any limitations to keep in mind and help create a customized plan based on your goals.

The American Heart Association recommends at least 150 minutes of moderate exercise, or 75 minutes of vigorous exercise, per week. If you're not used to that level of activity, start slow and build up your strength and endurance over time. This can help prevent injury.

Getting into a new routine and starting new habits can be challenging. Try the following:
- Set a reasonable goal: having a concrete but achievable goal in mind, like running a 5K or walking a certain number of steps per day, can help with motivation.
- Try different workouts: prevent boredom by trying different types of exercise, like tennis, group fitness classes, yoga, or weightlifting.
- Make it easy: setting out your workout clothes, shoes, and water bottle ahead of time can make it easier to establish these new habits.
- Remember the long-term: you might not see the rewards right away, but try to focus on the long-term rewards of feeling stronger, having more energy, and improving your health.

Tea is packed with phytonutrients (plant chemicals) called flavonoids, which have been shown to reduce inflammation and buildup in your arteries. Black and green tea also contain more moderate amounts of caffeine than coffee (about half the amount per cup), so tea is a great option for people who are sensitive to that.

ASCVD Risk Factors
- Cigarette smoking
- Hypertension
- Atherosclerosis of coronary arteries with stenosis
- Obesity
- Diabetes mellitus
- Sedentary lifestyle

Patients with no other apparent cardiovascular risk factors can still be at risk from elevated Lipoprotein(a) Lp(a).

Because elevated Lp(a) is an independent cardiovascular risk factor, an Lp(a) test may lead to a reclassification of patients otherwise considered at lower risk for cardiovascular disease.

A standard lipid panel does not distinguish Lp(a) from Low density lipoprotein LDL-C.

Lp(a) test can help delineate statin therapy goals.

Why Did the UK Ban Statins?

The controversy in the United Kingdom started in 2013 when the *British Medical Journal* (*BMJ*) claimed statins were being overprescribed to people with low risk of heart disease, and that the drugs' side effects were worse than previously thought.

Patients with Atherosclerosis

It is now accepted as a standard of care to lower LDL to less than 100 mg/dL in patients with atherosclerosis. Given the relatively small number of CHD patients with untreated LDL below this level and poor physician compliance with NCEP guidelines, and considering that non-LDL effects of statins may confer additional protection, the use of statins in all patients with atherosclerosis should be considered. Treatment in these patients should be initiated at the earliest opportunity, such as the time of diagnosis of an acute coronary or cerebrovascular event.

Patients with Diabetes

The risk of a major coronary event is as high in diabetic subjects without known CHD as in non-diabetic survivors of myocardial infarction. Data from studies show that the absolute risk reduction induced by statin treatment was larger in diabetic than in non-diabetic subjects. For this reason, LDL lowering is now recognized as the first priority in the control of diabetic dyslipidemia, and statin treatment should be implemented in the majority of type 2 diabetic patients with LDL of less than 100 mg/dL.

Asymptomatic Patients with Multiple Risk Factors

Statin therapy should be prioritized according to the patient's global risk. It is evident that among asymptomatic individuals, the absolute benefit of therapy with statins is greatest for subjects with the highest baseline risk. Statin therapy is highly recommended if the expected risk reduction is approximately 30 percent. Along this line of thinking, statins may be seen as antiatherogenic agents that will affect overall CHD risk even when the LDL level is not the most prominent problem within the risk profile.

Patients with Moderate Hypertriglyceridemia or Combined Hyperlipidemia

A recent consensus statement advocates the use of statins as first-line treatment in high-risk patients with triglyceride levels below 500 mg/dL. The combination of low-dose statin with nicotinic acid or fibrates for combined hyperlipidemia is a safe approach when performed with appropriate monitoring and after careful patient education. Statins are not appropriate first-line therapy in individuals with severe hypertriglyceridemia.

Patients with Low HDL

Data show impressive clinical benefits in subgroups with low levels of HDL. These results suggest that statin treatment may be appropriate for patients with low HDL levels not simply because of the LDL lowering and direct arterial wall effects but possibly also because of the increase in HDL. Given the combined effect of statins on LDL and HDL, it is reasonable to use the ratio of total cholesterol to HDL, as recommended by the Canadian guidelines, with a goal of less than 5 in high-risk and less than 4 in very-high-risk individuals.

Future Directions

Within the next few years, we will learn whether statins produce a benefit in the setting of acute coronary syndromes and how statin therapy, alone or as a major component of medical therapy, compares with revascularization procedures for patients with stable coronary disease. Indeed, a recent trial found that high-dose atorvastatin was at least as effective as angioplasty plus usual care in reducing coronary events in patients with stable CHD. Another important area of inquiry will be the evaluation of statin therapy in the prevention of stroke in subjects at high risk for cerebrovascular events.

Although statins are cost-effective in high-risk groups, they are vastly underutilized among patients with coronary disease. It is critically important that practices become organized so that high-risk patients are systematically identified and treated. Risk assessment is equally important to identify patients at the lower end of the risk spectrum, when the cost of statin therapy may not be justified.

Our understanding of the pharmacological effects of statins is evolving toward the realization that these agents do more than simply lower cholesterol. Similar to the ACE inhibitors, whose role as antihypertensive agents is now surpassed by their effects on cardiac and renal function, statins may produce benefits both by decreasing cholesterol and by lipid-independent mechanisms, and they are poised to become invaluable tools in the prevention and management of cardiovascular disease.

Rosuvastatin (Crestor) is commonly used to lower bad cholesterol levels (LDL-C) and fats (triglycerides) in the blood. It also increases good cholesterol levels (HDL). Improving your cholesterol levels helps decrease your risk of heart disease, stroke, and heart attack.

Very rarely, high-dose statin use can cause muscle cells to break down and release a protein called myoglobin into the bloodstream. This can lead to severe muscle pain, kidney damage, and liver damage.

Vitamin D supplements may have moderate or no effect on the dosage requirements or side effects of pravastatin, rosuvastatin, and pitavastatin. Since vitamin D has mild HMG-CoA reductase activity, it will work synergistically with all statins.

The verdict, according to the National Institutes of Health, is that there's insufficient evidence to determine any relationship between your vitamin D intake and your cholesterol levels.

Optimal vitamin K2 intake is crucial to avoid the calcium plaque buildup of atherosclerosis, thus keeping the risk and rate of calcification as low as possible. Matrix GLA protein (MGP)—found in the tissues of the heart, kidneys, and lungs—plays a dominant role in vascular calcium metabolism.

Surgical Options

CABG Surgery with Sephanous Vein graft and prior Myocardial Damage

If medicine or lifestyle changes don't work to treat a heart condition related to ASCVD, you may need surgery. Your surgeon may perform coronary artery bypass grafting (CABG). During this procedure, they'll redirect veins or arteries around narrowed coronary arteries from different parts of your body. The average cost of bypass surgery in the United States in 2020 was $30,000 to $200,000.

Treatment for coronary artery disease may also require surgical intervention, such as with angioplasty, stent replacement, coronary artery bypass graft surgery (CABG), or off-pump coronary artery bypass surgery.

There is no fast, easy way to unclog an artery once plaque has built up. However, following a heart-healthy eating plan; staying physically active, such as by regularly exercising; and quitting smoking (if you smoke) can help stop blockages from getting worse. In some cases, medications may be needed. Surgery to remove plaques or bypass the blockages, including cardiac bypass surgery, angioplasty and/or stent replacement, weight-loss surgery, and carotid endarterectomy may be recommended also.

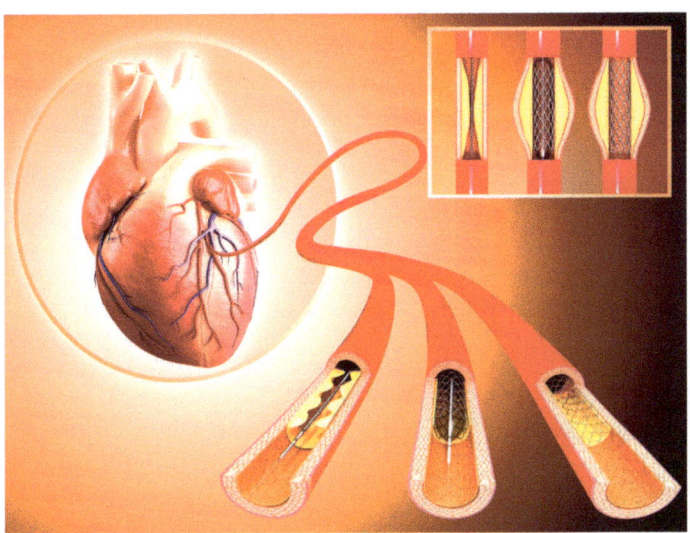

Coronary Angioplasty and Stent Placement

Complications
If you have clogged arteries, working with a doctor to create a treatment plan is essential. If blockages remain untreated, you could experience severe health complications, including angina, coronary artery disease, coronary microvascular disease, heart attack, carotid artery disease, stroke, peripheral vascular disease (PVD), and chronic kidney disease (CKD).

Following a heart-healthy diet, staying physically active, and quitting smoking (if you smoke) may help reduce plaque buildup and stop blockages from getting worse. If lifestyle changes are not enough, a doctor may prescribe medication, such as statins, to help lower your LDL cholesterol and prevent plaque formation.

Takeaway
Plaque buildup may clog your arteries. Though diet and lifestyle are major contributors to arterial blockages, your risk of atherosclerosis may also increase with age.

Adopting a heart-healthy eating plan and staying physically active, such as by exercising regularly, may help reduce plaques and prevent them from getting worse. These health-promoting lifestyle changes are also essential if you have a procedure to remove plaques or bypass a heavily clogged artery.

If you have questions about clogged arteries, talk with a health-care professional.

Magnesium supplementation can inhibit atherosclerotic plaque formation in animals on high-fat diets. More recent human studies have revealed strong associations between low magnesium levels and higher heart disease risks. This demonstrates that magnesium can be a powerful protective measure to maintain heart health.

Chelation therapy is hyped as a way to clean out the arteries by dissolving cholesterol-filled plaque. This is based on wishful thinking, not science. Apple cider vinegar is a terrific ingredient in foods, sauces, and dressings. It isn't medicine.

Fruits such as strawberries and mulberries contain a lot of antioxidant flavonoids, which work to clean the plaque that is forming and prevent hardening of the arteries. Therefore, it can be affirmed that mulberry fruit is an effective blood-vessel-cleaning food.

A traditional Mediterranean diet with added olive oil may be tied to a lower risk of heart disease at least in part because it helps maintain healthy blood flow and clear debris from arteries, a Spanish study suggests.

From a broad perspective, eating a diet rich in anti-inflammatory, antioxidant-rich foods (think veggies, low-glycemic fruits, nuts, seeds, fish, olive oil), scaling way back on sugar, and swapping out refined grains like bread for small quantities of whole grains like quinoa is helpful. The drug trodusquemine can be used to reverse the effects of a buildup of fat inside the arteries of mice; researchers have published new findings demonstrating the same positive results.

Bright red cayenne pepper does more than just spice up your food. Thanks to a compound called capsaicin, cayenne pepper can help your arteries work well. It can also help relax the muscles in your blood vessels so blood can flow easily. And that's good for your blood pressure.

Ginger, pepper, chili, and cinnamon are all anti-inflammatory spices and help in improving blood lipid levels and keeping arteries clear.

Foods high in potassium, like bananas, can stop fatal blockages from occurring and inhibit the hardening and narrowing of arteries.

Eating oats can help significantly reduce atherosclerosis risk factors, including high total and LDL (bad) cholesterol. Oats also contain antioxidants called avenanthramides, which may help inhibit inflammatory proteins called cytokines and adhesion molecules.

The following fruits are associated with numerous health benefits, including the ability to reduce inflammation and improve heart health: blueberries, strawberries, cranberries, raspberries, and mulberries. Berries contain fiber, vitamins, minerals, and beneficial plant compounds. These include flavonoid antioxidants, including polyphenols, which may support heart health.

Eating beans is an excellent way to manage cholesterol levels, reducing your risk of clogged arteries. Many studies have demonstrated that eating beans can significantly reduce LDL (bad) cholesterol levels. Beans offer various cardioprotective effects, including reducing blood pressure, reducing blood triglyceride levels, lowering LDL and total cholesterol levels, reducing inflammation, and improving artery function.

Bean-rich diets can also improve insulin sensitivity, body weight and waist circumference, colon health, and gut microbiome diversity.

All these effects may reduce the risk of atherosclerosis.

Eating omega-3-rich fish may help reduce the risk of atherosclerosis and coronary artery disease, though researchers have not yet definitively determined why.

Onions are part of the *Allium* genus and are linked to health benefits, including supporting artery health. Research has shown that a diet rich in these popular veggies may protect the arteries. Onions contain sulfur compounds that scientists think may help prevent blood vessel inflammation, inhibit the clumping together of platelets in the blood, and increase the availability of nitric oxide. All these effects may help protect against atherosclerosis and improve artery health.

Citrus fruits are delicious and provide a variety of vitamins, minerals, and antioxidants, including flavonoids.

Citrus flavonoids can decrease inflammation and help prevent free radicals in the body from oxidizing LDL (bad) cholesterol. Oxidized LDL is associated with atherosclerosis development and progression. This may be why citrus consumption is associated with a reduced risk of heart disease and stroke—two conditions linked to atherosclerosis.

Spices, including ginger, pepper, chili, and cinnamon, may help protect against clogged arteries. These and other spices have anti-inflammatory properties and may help reduce free radicals, improve blood lipid levels, and reduce the clumping together of platelets in the blood. You can increase your spice consumption by adding these versatile flavorings to oatmeal, soups, stews, and just about any other dish you can think of.

One serving of flaxseed provides protein, fiber, and omega-3 fatty acids. It may help lower the risk of some cancers, help you maintain a moderate weight, and reduce cholesterol and blood pressure.

Eating certain foods may help prevent clogged arteries and lower your risk of heart disease. Some examples include berries, beans, tomatoes, fish, oats, and leafy greens.

Green tea may lower your cholesterol if you are an avid tea drinker. For your heart health, it pays to go green. Powerful antioxidants in green tea—especially one called epigallocatechin gallate, or EGCG, can help prevent atherosclerosis and plaque buildup in the arteries.

The following are some healthy breakfast choices for clogged arteries: Scrambled eggs, whole-grain toast, one cup of milk and sliced apples. Greek yogurt with whole-grain cereal and berries. Whole-grain toast with peanut butter or alternative, sliced apples, one cup of milk. Yogurt parfait with plain yogurt, ground flax seeds or muesli, and fresh fruit.

Lifestyle factors such as a healthy diet rich in fruits and vegetables, regular exercise, and not smoking are well-known remedies for improving heart health.

Those individuals who practiced intermittent fasting also had about 40 percent less atherosclerosis in their carotid arteries than the control group.

Peanut butter also contains omega-6 fatty acid. This fatty acid lowers bad (LDL) cholesterol and increases good (HDL) cholesterol. In addition, peanuts are a natural source of arginine, an amino acid that may prevent heart and vascular disease by promoting good blood vessel function.

Among the different supplements that claim to promote heart health, there are four that have relatively more evidence supporting them. Omega-3 fatty acids may lower inflammation in the body, which may reduce certain risk factors linked to heart disease. Folate (vitamin B9), vitamin D, and magnesium are also recommended.

Making plaque disappear is not possible, but with lifestyle changes and medication, plaque deposits can shrink and stabilize.

Water fasting has been linked with some impressive health benefits, including a lower risk of certain cancers, heart disease, and diabetes. Water fasting may also promote autophagy, a process in which your body breaks down and recycles old, potentially dangerous parts of your cells.

Garlic may help lower high blood pressure; it may also help prevent the scarring and hardening associated with atherosclerosis. Some research has also shown that aged garlic extract can help reduce the amount of "soft plaque" in the arteries.

Walnuts are rich in alphalinoleic acid, which has anti-inflammatory properties and has been shown to help reduce plaque buildup in coronary arteries and thus lower your risk for developing heart disease.

Pistachios are packed with nutrients such as protein while also low in calories and low in fats. This makes them a great option if you are looking to lose or maintain your weight, as eating them can help you feel full for longer. Pistachios can thus help you reduce your chances of developing obesity, which is a major risk factor for heart disease.

The worst foods for high cholesterol, given their high saturated fat content, include the following: red meat like beef, pork, and sausage; full-fat dairy, like cream, whole milk, and butter; baked goods, sweets, fried foods, and tropical oils such as palm oil and coconut oil.

There is some evidence that CoQ10 may help treat heart failure when combined with conventional medications. People who have congestive heart failure, where the heart is not able to pump blood as well as it should, may also have low levels of CoQ10.

Lipitor can clean out plaque in your arteries. There have been several clinical studies that show statins can reverse plaque buildup. Two statins in particular, atorvastatin, which is sold under the brand name Lipitor, and rosuvastatin, which is sold under the brand name Crestor, are the strongest statins.

Cinnamaldehyde, an organic compound in cinnamon, has also been shown to have anticoagulant properties that may help curb the risk of blood clots, and preliminary research suggests that cinnamon inhibits the atherosclerosis process in animals with high cholesterol.

Bananas contain fiber, potassium, folate, and antioxidants, such as vitamin C. All these support heart health. A 2017 review found that people who follow a high-fiber diet have a lower risk of cardiovascular disease than those on a low-fiber diet.

Golden milk, also known as turmeric milk, is a common Indian drink that has recently been gaining popularity in Western cultures due to many health claims. Its beautiful bright yellow color is a result of adding turmeric, along with spices such as cinnamon and ginger, to milk.

CEREBROVASCULAR ACCIDENTS (CVAS): STROKES AND TRANSIENT ISCHEMIC ATTACKS (TIAS)

Globally, one in four people over age twenty-five will have a stroke in their lifetime. Each year, over 16 percent of all strokes occur in people fifteen to forty-nine years of age. Each year, over 62 percent of all strokes occur in people under seventy years of age.

Incidence and Risk Factors

The American Heart Association notes that annually more than 795,000 people in the United States have a stroke. An estimated 610,000 of these are first or new strokes, with 185,000 people experiencing subsequent strokes within five years.

While the incidence of stroke is decreasing overall in this country, rates among young adults are increasing. Roughly 800,000 Americans suffer strokes each year. While only 15 percent of strokes occur in those aged eighteen to fifty, 120,000 Americans under fifty and 1.5 million young adults worldwide suffer strokes each year.

The incidence rate of first-ever stroke in China (505.2 per 100,000 person-years) was higher than that in Japan (317.0 per

100,000 person-years for ages forty-five and older), Singapore (229.6 per 100,000), and the European Union (67 per 100,000).

The number of people who will die from strokes worldwide is likely to rise 50 percent by 2050, with ten million people dying from stroke yearly. Currently, fifteen million people globally have a stroke each year.

The number one cause of stroke in the United States is cigarette smoking.

Blockage of the carotid artery is the leading cause of stroke in Americans. Also, nicotine raises blood pressure, carbon monoxide from smoking reduces the amount of oxygen your blood can carry to your brain, and cigarette smoke makes your blood thicker and more likely to clot.

Having an irregular heartbeat (atrial fibrillation) is the most powerful and treatable heart risk factor of stroke.

African Americans are 50 percent more likely to have a stroke (cerebrovascular disease) as compared to their white adult counterparts.

Some rare conditions can predispose some people to stroke at a young age. But most risk factors for stroke in young adults are similar to those in older adults: high blood pressure, diabetes, high cholesterol, and obesity. These conditions are becoming more and more common among younger Americans.

Some people will experience symptoms such as headache, numbness, or tingling several days before they have a serious stroke. One study found that 43 percent of stroke patients experienced ministroke symptoms up to a week before they had a major stroke.

You might have heard the FAST acronym before. It's an easy way to remember the most common warning signs of a stroke and the importance of acting quickly:

- Face drooping (if you ask the person to smile, then it will be crooked or one-sided)

- Arm weakness or numbness (if you ask the person to lift both arms, one will drop lower than the other)
- Speech problems such as slurring or difficulty repeating a sentence
- Time to call an ambulance

However, there are some other possible symptoms that you should watch out for too:

- A sudden, severe headache
- Sudden dizziness, loss of balance, or coordination
- Loss of vision or changes to vision in one or both eyes, which usually happens suddenly
- Feeling confused or having trouble understanding things that are usually easy for you
- Numbness or weakness on one side of the body (or in one arm or leg)

The signs of a stroke often appear suddenly, but that doesn't mean that you won't have time to act. If you think that you or another person might be having a TIA or stroke, then you need to get help right away. A stroke is a medical emergency, so the faster you get treatment, the better. Call an ambulance right away and tell the paramedics that you suspect a stroke. Remember that you still need to go to hospital if the symptoms disappear, as it may have been a ministroke.

The treatment you're given will depend on the type of stroke, the area of the brain that is affected, and how severe the symptoms are. The first priority will be to restore the blood supply to your brain. It might be possible to dissolve a blood clot using medicine, but sometimes a surgical procedure is required. The sooner that you get this treatment, the better the results.

Once the immediate threat has been treated, you will probably need longer-term treatment to prevent more strokes and to help you recover. You might need medication to prevent clots from forming or to reduce your blood pressure. Sometimes surgery is recommended to improve the blood supply to the brain. You might need extra support to manage any long-term effects such as speech or mobility problems. The sooner you get help, the easier it will be to treat you and the less likely you will be to experience long-term effects.

If your blood pressure is very high, seek medical care. Call 911 or emergency medical services if your blood pressure is 180/120 mm Hg or greater and you have chest pain, shortness of breath, or symptoms of stroke.

A high blood pressure reading above 130/80 mm Hg can increase the risk of stroke. Elevated blood pressure can cause various physiological changes, such as damage to the blood vessels of the brain and bleeding in the brain. These changes can cause ischemic or hemorrhagic strokes or strokes due to small-vessel disease.

Even higher blood pressure (with the systolic blood pressure 180 or higher, the diastolic blood pressure more than 120, or both) is called a hypertensive urgency if there are no related symptoms. Or it's called a hypertensive emergency if there are symptoms indicating damage to the brain, heart, or kidneys.

A type of stroke occurs when a blood clot or fatty plaque blocks a blood vessel in the brain. Symptoms include drooping muscles on one side of the face and numbness or weakness on one side of the face or in one arm or leg. Treatment includes medications, medical procedures, and surgical procedures. These will be elaborated later.

The stroke belt is typically defined to include the states of Alabama, Arkansas, Georgia, Kentucky, Louisiana, Mississippi, North Carolina, South Carolina, Tennessee, and Virginia. These eleven states had an age-adjusted stroke mortality rate of 10 percent.

From 2019 to 2021, Mississippi had the highest rate of death due to stroke of any US state, with around fifty-five deaths per 100,000 people.

Some research suggests coffee can lower the risk of high blood pressure, also called hypertension, in people who don't already have it. But drinking too much coffee has been shown to raise blood pressure and lead to anxiety, heart palpitations, and trouble sleeping.

COVID-19 is known to increase the risk of heart attack and stroke. The intense inflammation that occurs throughout the body in severe cases likely contributes to this increased risk.

In comparison with Western populations, stroke in Asians appears more likely due to small-vessel (lacunar) disease, intracranial athero-occlusive stenosis, and spontaneous intracerebral hemorrhage.

Over twelve million people worldwide will have their first stroke this year, and 6.5 million will die as a result. Over 100 million people in the world have experienced stroke. The incidence of stroke increases significantly with age; however, over 60 percent of strokes happen to people under the age of seventy, and 16 percent happen to those under the age of fifty.

Over half of people who have a stroke will die as a result. For survivors the impact can be devastating: strokes affect physical mobility, eating, speech and language, emotions, and thought processes. These complex needs can result in care and financial challenges for the individual and for their caregivers, as well as placing significant demands on health and social welfare provision.

Rates of stroke are growing fastest in low- and middle-income countries, where health-care providers often find it more challenging to provide the care that is needed for effective prevention, treatment, and rehabilitation of stroke.

Conclusions

In 2016, the global lifetime risk of stroke from the age of twenty-five years onward was approximately 25 percent among both men and women. There was geographic variation in the lifetime risk of stroke, with the highest risks in East Asia, central Europe, and eastern Europe.

Stroke accounts for almost 5 percent of all disability-adjusted life-years and 10 percent of all deaths worldwide, with the bulk of this burden (more than 75 percent of deaths from stroke and more than 80 percent of disability-adjusted life-years) occurring in low-income and middle-income countries. According to several surveys, the global burden of stroke has been increasing, and prevention of stroke may require an improved understanding of the risks among younger persons.

Stroke prevention strategies in low-income and middle-income countries may differ from those adopted in high-income countries owing to differences in access to health care, health technologies, and relative rates of risk factors for stroke.

Estimates of lifetime risk (defined as the cumulative probability of a disease developing in a person of a given age and sex during that person's remaining lifespan, after accounting for competing risks of death) provide a measure of disease risk in large populations.

Estimates of lifetime risk of stroke may be useful for the long-term planning of health systems. In addition, estimates of lifetime risk of stroke across the age spectrum on a national level may be useful for gauging the effect of stroke prevention strategies.

Previous estimates of lifetime risk of stroke have been reported in a limited number of selected populations.

Diverging trends in stroke incidence and mortality rates have been observed between developed countries (where the rates are decreasing) and developing countries (where the rates are increasing) against a background of increasing life expectancy in almost all countries.

The Global Burden of Disease (GBD) Study 2016 estimated major disease burden from 1990 through 2016 to compare the estimated global, regional, and country-specific lifetime risks of stroke in 2016 with those in 1990. These estimates were stratified according to pathological subtype of stroke, age, sex, and sociodemographic index (SDI) and accounted for the competing risk of death from any cause other than stroke.

The GBD is an ongoing global collaboration that uses all available epidemiologic data to provide a comparative assessment of health loss from 328 diseases across 195 countries and territories.

The global economic impact of stroke currently represents 0.66 percent of global GDP, and the total cost of stroke is expected to tip US $1 trillion by 2030.

The estimated global cost of stroke is over $721 billion (0.66 percent of global GDP).

Risk Factors

Risk factors for stroke include the following:
- Tobacco smoking
- Hypertension
- Diabetes mellitus
- Carotid atherosclerosis with stenosis
- Atrial fibrillation with cerebral embolism
- PFO with cerebral embolism
- Sedentary lifestyle

Treatment Options

Preventing stroke is critically important.

Treatment consists of blood thinners. Early treatment with medications like tPA (a clot buster) can minimize brain damage. Other treatments focus on limiting complications and preventing additional strokes:
- Alteplase: can treat blood clots.

- Anticoagulants: prevent unwanted reactions from taking drugs that inhibit blood clotting. The most common problem is too much bleeding, which can be very serious.
- Statins: decrease the liver's production of harmful cholesterol.
- Antihypertensive drugs: lower blood pressure.
- ACE inhibitors: relax blood vessels, lower blood pressure, and prevent diabetes-related kidney damage.

The main treatment for an ischemic stroke is a medicine called tissue plasminogen activator (tPA). It breaks up the blood clots that block blood flow to your brain. A health-care provider will inject tPA into a vein in your arm. This type of medicine must be given within three hours after stroke symptoms start.

Administering tPA quickly dissolves the clots that cause many strokes. By opening a blocked blood vessel and restoring blood flow, tPA can reduce the amount of damage to the brain that can occur during a stroke. To be effective, tPA and other drugs like it must be given within a few hours of the stroke symptoms beginning.

How do medical professionals stop a stroke in progress? Staff in the emergency department will administer acute stroke medications to try to stop a stroke while it is happening. Ischemic stroke, the most common type of stroke, is treated with the "clot-busting" drug known as tPA.

What is the golden hour for stroke? People who arrive within the first hour are more likely to receive tissue plasminogen activator (tPA)—the only proven treatment for acute ischemic stroke—than are those who arrive between one and three hours after onset.

Remember that the warning signs of stroke include weakness or numbness of the face, arm, or leg, usually on one side of the body; trouble speaking or understanding; and problems with vision, such as dimness or loss of vision in one or both eyes.

The signs and symptoms of a stroke often occur quickly. However, they can develop over hours or even days. This sometimes happens when a transient ischemic attack (TIA)—a blockage that breaks up before it damages your brain—turns into a stroke.

After an initial assessment, you will be referred to a specialist for further tests to help determine the cause of the stroke. You should be referred to see a specialist within twenty-four hours of the start of your symptoms. Treatment can also begin if necessary.

It means you're at an increased risk of having a stroke in the near future.

It's important to call 911 immediately and ask for an ambulance if you or someone else has TIA or stroke symptoms.

If a TIA is suspected, you will be offered aspirin to take right away. This helps to prevent a stroke.

Even if the symptoms disappear while you're waiting for the ambulance to arrive, an assessment in a hospital should still be done.

If you think you have had a TIA before, but the symptoms have since passed and you did not get medical advice at the time, make an urgent appointment with your primary care provider. Your primary care provider can refer you for a hospital assessment, if appropriate.

Call 911 or emergency medical services if your blood pressure is 180/120 mm Hg or greater and you have chest pain, shortness of breath, or symptoms of stroke. Stroke symptoms include numbness or tingling, trouble speaking, or changes in vision.

When a stroke affects the emotion center of the brain, it can cause a condition called the pseudo-bulbar affect. This involves involuntary, inappropriate, and uncontrollable outbursts of emotion such as laughter, crying, or anger, particularly when a situation does not call for such emotion.

Normal pressure is 120/80 or lower. Your blood pressure is considered high (stage 1) if it reads 130/80 to 139/89. Stage 2 high blood pressure is 140/90 or higher. If you get a blood pressure reading of 180/120 or higher more than once, seek medical treatment right away.

Changes in your emotions and to your personality are common after stroke. It's very normal to experience strong emotions after stroke; however, these emotional reactions usually get better with time. Longer-term emotional and personality changes can be very challenging.

Surgical Treatment of Carotid Stenosis: Carotid Endarterectomy

Carotid endarterectomy is a surgical procedure used to reduce the risk of stroke from carotid artery stenosis (narrowing of the internal carotid artery).

In endarterectomy, the surgeon opens the artery and removes the plaque. The plaque forms and thickens the inner layer of the artery, or intima—hence the name of the procedure, which simply means removal of part of the internal layers of the artery.

The carotid endarterectomy specimen is removed from within the lumen of the common carotid artery (bottom), and the internal carotid artery (left) and external carotid artery (right).

An alternative procedure is carotid stenting, which can also reduce the risk of stroke for some patients.

Carotid endarterectomy is used to reduce the risk of strokes caused by carotid artery stenosis over time. Carotid stenosis can either have symptoms (i.e., be symptomatic) or be found by a doctor in the absence of symptoms (asymptomatic), and the risk reduction from endarterectomy is greater for symptomatic than asymptomatic patients.

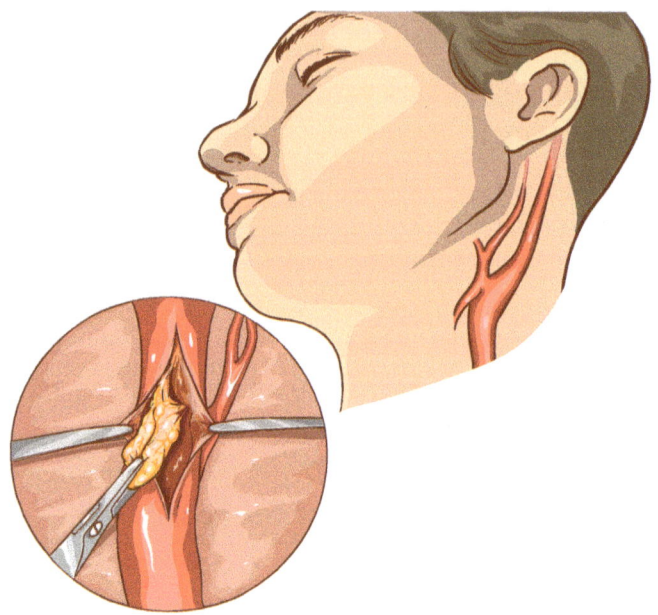

Carotid Endarterectomy

Carotid endarterectomy itself can cause strokes, so for this procedure to be of benefit in preventing strokes over time, the risks for combined thirty-day mortality and stroke risk following surgery should be less than 3 percent for asymptomatic people and less than or equal to 6 percent for symptomatic people.

Carotid endarterectomy does not treat symptoms of prior strokes. It is controversial if carotid endarterectomy can improve cognitive function in some patients.

Symptomatic people have had either a stroke or a transient ischemic attack.

In symptomatic patients with a 70 to 99 percent stenosis, for every six people treated, one major stroke would be prevented at two years.

Unlike asymptomatic patients, symptomatic people with moderate carotid stenosis (50 to 69 percent) still benefit from endarterectomy, albeit to a lesser degree. In addition, comorbidity adversely affects the outcome: people with multiple medical problems have a higher postoperative mortality rate and hence benefit less from the procedure. For maximum benefit people should be operated on soon after a stroke or transient ischemic attack, preferably within the first two weeks.

Asymptomatic people have narrowing of their carotid arteries but have not experienced a transient ischemic attack or stroke. The annual risk of stroke in patients with asymptomatic carotid disease is between 1 percent and 2 percent, although some patients are considered to be at higher risk, such as those with ulcerated plaques. This low rate of stroke means that there is less potential stroke risk reduction from endarterectomy for asymptomatic patients relative to symptomatic patients. However, for asymptomatic patients with severe carotid stenosis (80 to 99 percent), carotid endarterectomy plus treatment with a statin medicine and antiplatelet therapy does reduce stroke risk further than medication alone in the five years following surgery.

Carotid Artery Stenting

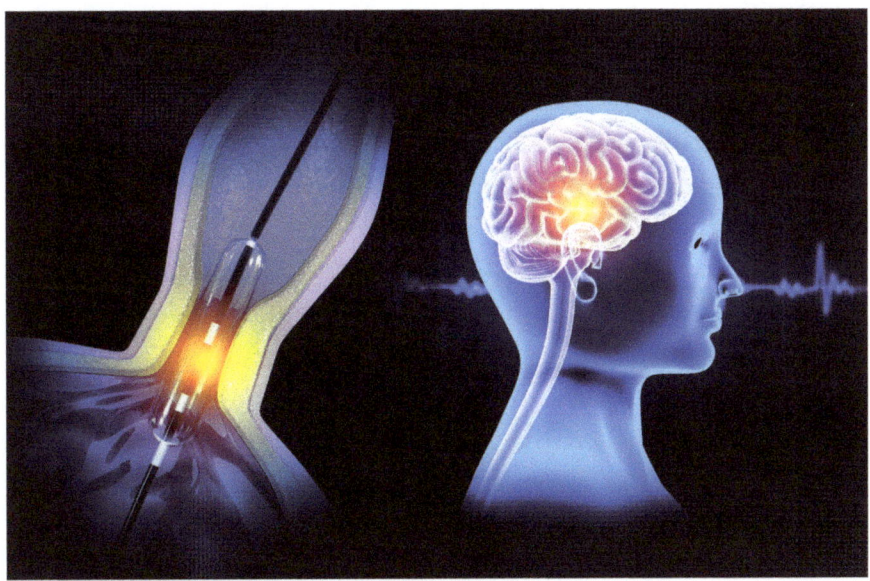

Carotid Balloon Angioplasty with stent Placement

Carotid artery stenting is an endovascular procedure where a stent is deployed within the lumen of the carotid artery to treat narrowing of the carotid artery and decrease the risk of stroke. It is used to treat narrowing of the carotid artery in high-risk patients, when carotid endarterectomy is considered too risky.

Carotid stenting is used to reduce the risk of stroke associated with carotid artery stenosis. Carotid stenosis can have no symptoms or have symptoms such as transient ischemic attacks (TIAs) or strokes.

While historically endarterectomy has been the treatment for carotid stenosis, stenting is an alternative intervention for patients who are not candidates for surgery.

High risk factors for endarterectomy that would favor stenting instead include medical co-morbidities such as severe heart disease, heart failure, severe lung disease, and anatomic features (contralateral carotid occlusion, radiation therapy to the neck, prior ipsilateral carotid artery surgery, intra-thoracic or intracranial carotid disease) that would make surgery difficult and risky.

While rates of stroke and death after both surgery and stenting are low, rates of stroke and death after stenting may be higher than those after endarterectomy, particularly for transfemoral stenting in patients over age seventy.

Carotid stenting involves the placement of a stent across the stenosis in the carotid artery. It can be performed under general or local anesthesia.

The stent may be placed from the femoral artery, from the radial artery, or from the common carotid artery at the base of the neck. Critical steps in both approaches are vascular access, crossing the stenosis with a wire, deploying a stent across the lesion, and removing the vascular access. A number of other steps may or may not be performed, including the use of a cerebral protection device, pre- or post-stent balloon, angioplasty, and cerebral angiography.

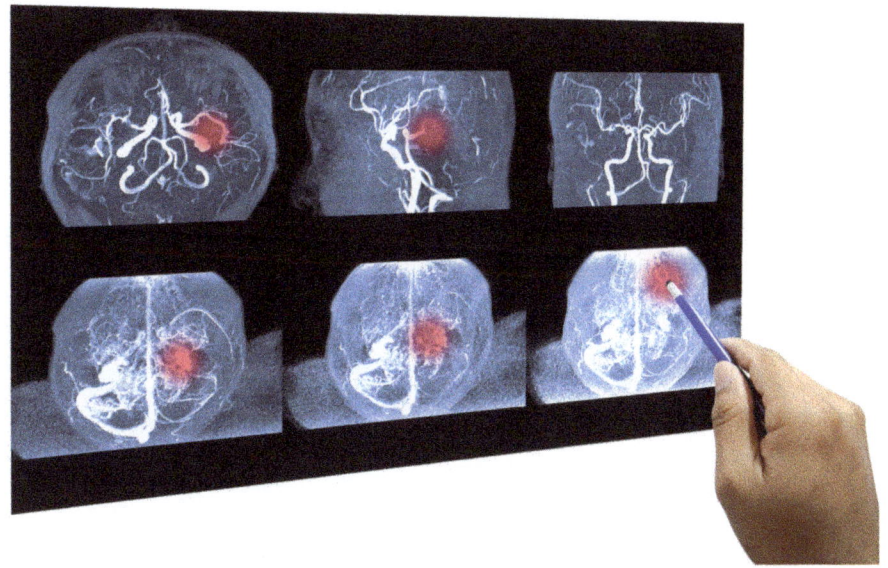

Magnetic Resonance Angiography (MRA) of Cerebral Vessels

The trans-femoral route is the traditional approach to carotid stenting. The vast majority of these procedures are performed under local anesthesia. In this technique, puncture of the common femoral artery is used to gain access to the arterial system. A wire and sheath are advanced through the aorta to the common carotid artery on the side to be treated. Flow reversal or filter cerebral protection may be used. The procedure is typically performed percutaneously.

Trans-carotid artery stenting involves a surgical incision at the base of the neck over the common carotid artery. It is performed under either local or general anesthesia. Wire access is obtained at that location and used to deliver the stent to the internal carotid artery. Cerebral protection is usually obtained by flow reversal—the common carotid artery is clamped, and arterial blood from the internal carotid is run through a filter and returned to a femoral vein during the highest risk of the procedure.

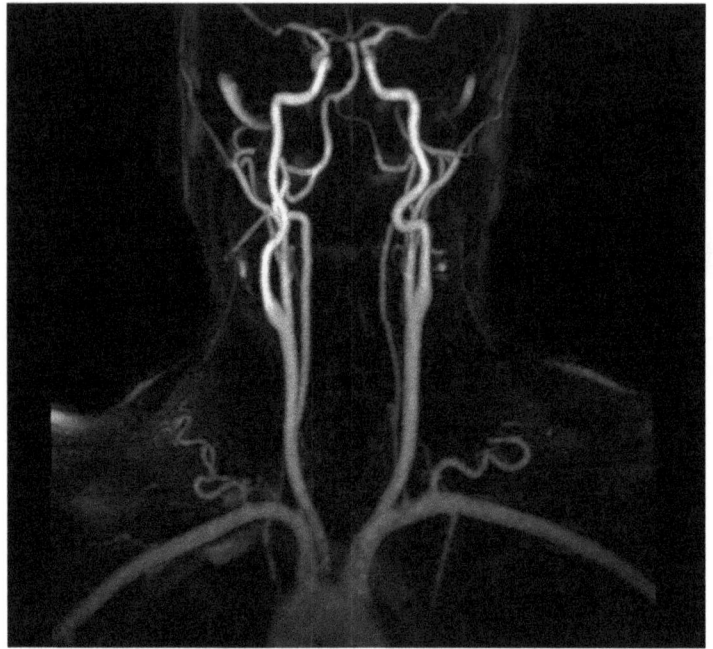

MRI Showing Carotid and Cerebral Arteries

The trans-radial route has been introduced as an alternative in the past few years. The vast majority of these procedures are performed under local anesthesia. In this technique, puncture of the radial artery is used to gain access to the arterial system. Again a wire and sheath are advanced through the aorta to the common carotid artery on the side to be treated. Flow reversal or filter cerebral protection may be used. The procedure is typically performed percutaneously.

Recovery after carotid artery stenting depends not only on the presence of complications during the procedure but also on the presence of symptoms at the time of arrival to the hospital. Asymptomatic patients typically leave the hospital in in a day or less. The blood pressure is kept at a goal below 140 mm Hg systolic. Elevated blood pressure two to ten days postoperatively may lead to reperfusion syndrome.

The most feared short-term complication of any stroke prevention procedure on the carotid artery is stroke itself. Patients must still be carefully selected for surgery or stenting in order to reduce the risks related to the procedure and ensure a long-term benefit after such intervention. Other short-term complications might include bleeding, infection, and heart problems such as myocardial infarction related to anesthesia.

Late complications such as recurrent stenosis may occur, and surveillance with duplex ultrasound or CT angiography may be performed.

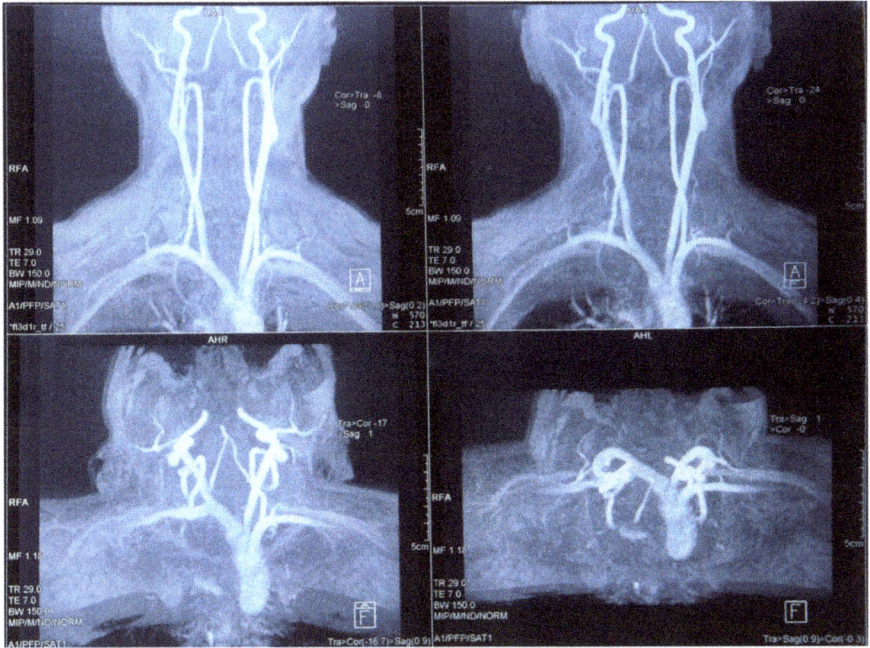

CT of Carotid Arteries

The risk reduction from intervention for carotid stenosis (stenting or endarterectomy) is greatest when the indication for intervention is symptoms (i.e., the patient is symptomatic)–typically stroke or TIA.

A new generation of double-layer stents is currently being developed to reduce the risk of stroke during or after the procedure. There is insufficient evidence to say that stenting or endarterectomy is better for symptomatic patients.

Angioplasty and carotid stenting in patients with asymptomatic carotid atherosclerotic stenosis should not be performed except in the context of randomized clinical trials.

Post-stroke Brain Changes

Changes in your emotions and to your personality are common after stroke. It's very normal to experience strong emotions after stroke; however, these emotional reactions usually get better with time. Longer-term emotional and personality changes can be very challenging.

A stroke can damage parts of the brain that are linked to the emotions. Some people have difficulty controlling their moods and seem angry or irritable, which can put a strain on relationships. Some people find that they become more sexual or lose inhibitions. Although stroke survivors should be cautious about physical activity, sex is not considered a specific risk factor for another stroke.

When certain areas of the brain sustain tissue damage, this can cause a survivor to struggle with empathy or emotional regulation. As a result, a survivor may demonstrate behavior that seems self-centered or selfish after stroke.

After a stroke, survivors often experience a range of emotional and behavioral changes. The reason is simple. Stroke impacts the brain, and the brain controls our behavior and emotions. You or your loved one may experience feelings of irritability, forgetfulness, carelessness, inattention, or confusion.

Many people have problems with their memory after a stroke, especially in the first weeks and months. A stroke often affects short-term memory more than long-term.

Almost a quarter of people who have had a stroke will go on to develop dementia after about three to six months. Research to date has not been able to explain why some people develop dementia after stroke and others don't.

Sometimes, after a stroke, people are not able to recognize the effect that it has on them. You may not know that you've lost movement in your arm or leg, for example. This is called anosognosia.

Below are common types of cognitive problems after stroke:
- Concentration problems
- Memory problems
- Problems with planning and problem-solving (executive function)
- Problems noticing things on one side (spatial neglect)
- Problems moving or controlling your body (apraxia)
- Problems controlling movement and finding your way around (visual perception)

Vascular dementia is the second most common type of dementia behind Alzheimer's disease. It happens when the brain suffers an injury due to decreased blood flow. There are no approved medications for post-stroke dementia. Instead, doctors may recommend drugs used to treat other types of dementia.

Mental illnesses that are commonly associated with stroke are depression, anxiety, fatigue, sleep disturbances, and emotionalism.

Three major mental health disorders common after stroke include: (1) post-stroke depression, (2) post-stroke anxiety, and (3) post-traumatic stress disorder. Other associated disorders and concerns include psychosis, mania, and suicidal ideation.

Cognitive impairment or dementia after stroke is predominantly defined by dementia that occurred within three months after stroke onset. Regardless, many stroke survivors develop delayed dementia beyond three months or only after recurrent strokes.

Drinking enough water regularly prevents dehydration. This may play a role in keeping the blood less viscous, which in turn prevents a stroke. However, this does not mean over-hydration is a healthy habit. Drinking too much water may be dangerous too, especially in people with heart and kidney conditions.

INTERVENTIONAL THERAPY

Before you agree to the test or the procedure, make sure you know the following:
- The name of the test or procedure
- The reason you are having the test or procedure
- What results to expect and what they mean
- The risks and benefits of the test or procedure
- What the possible side effects or complications are
- When and where you are to have the test or procedure
- Who will do the test or procedure and what that person's qualifications are
- What would happen if you did not have the test or procedure
- Any alternative tests or procedures to think about
- When and how will you get the results
- Who to call after the test or procedure if you have questions or problems
- How much you will have to pay for the test or procedure

Coronary Angioplasty and Stents
Percutaneous transluminal coronary angioplasty (PTCA) is also known as coronary angioplasty. It is a type of percutaneous coronary intervention (PCI), or minimally invasive procedure, to correct clogged arteries.

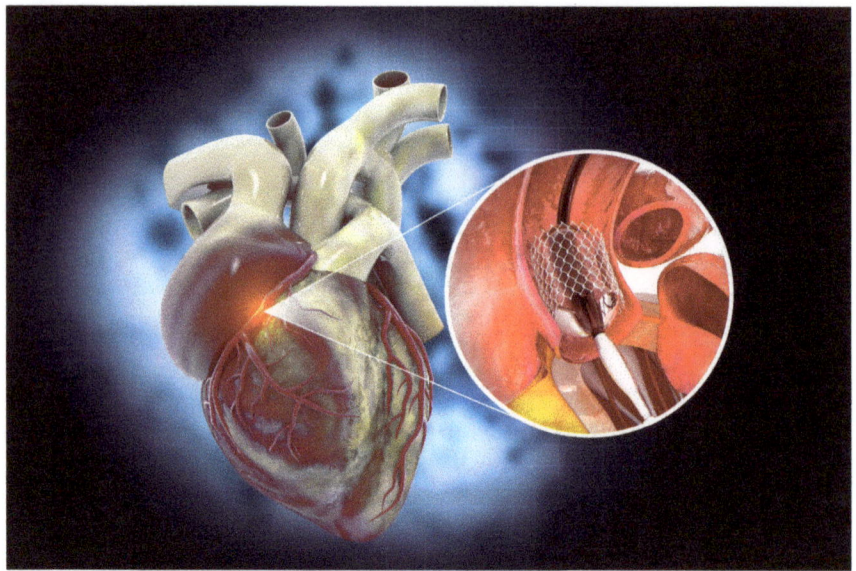

Coronary Balloon Angioplasty with Stent Placement

Coronary Artery Bypass Grafting (CABG) Surgery

Coronary artery bypass grafting (CABG), also called heart bypass surgery, is a medical procedure to improve blood flow to the heart. It may be needed when the arteries supplying blood to the heart, called coronary arteries, are narrowed or blocked.

CABG uses healthy blood vessels from another part of the body and connects them to blood vessels above and below the blocked artery. This creates a new route for blood flow that bypasses the narrowed or blocked coronary arteries. The blood vessels are usually arteries from the arm or chest, or veins from the legs.

In traditional "open-heart" CABG, your heart is stopped, and a heart-lung bypass machine takes over the job of pumping blood throughout the body. This is still the most common approach, but other techniques, called "off-pump" procedures because the heart does not need to be stopped, may be an option for some people.

As with any surgery, there are risks and possible complications. As part of your recovery from CABG surgery, your doctor may recommend medicines and heart-healthy lifestyle changes to further reduce your symptoms, treat your disease, and help prevent complications such as blood clots. Your doctor will also talk to you about steps you can take to prevent or lower your risk for future blockages or other problems.

If you have severe coronary artery disease, you are more likely to need coronary angioplasty or some type of CABG surgery. These treatments can help reduce chest pain and the risk of a heart attack as well as improve survival. It is possible that your type of blockages will not respond as well to treatment with angioplasty. In this case, you may need CABG surgery. Certain types of blockages may respond better to CABG than to angioplasty. For certain people one procedure or the other is clearly the best choice. Talk with your health-care provider about the risks and benefits of both. Also ask if you have any choice in which surgery to have.

Once you and your health-care provider have decided on CABG, you will need to decide what type of surgery is right for you. Certain types of people at high risk may be more likely to benefit from off-pump CABG. These include people with advanced atherosclerosis of the aorta, kidney problems, or chronic lung disease. Off-pump CABG may reduce the risks of postoperative inflammation, infection, and irregular heart rhythms. It is important to have off-pump CABG performed by a surgeon with experience in the approach. Different surgical centers and different surgeons may prefer one technique over the other. Ask your health-care provider about your risks and the benefits of CABG with or without a heart-lung machine.

On-Pump CABG Surgery

On-pump CABG is a time-honored procedure that is performed while the heart is stopped. The blood supply must be provided to the rest of the body when the heart is stopped.

Off-Pump CABG Surgery (Beating-Heart Surgery)

As discussed above, an "off-pump CABG" is a CABG performed without the use of a heart-lung machine (cardiopulmonary bypass). This means the heart continues to provide blood to the rest of the body during the surgery. It is sometimes referred to as "beating-heart surgery." In another method used during surgery, a machine takes over the functions of the heart and the lungs and the heart is still.

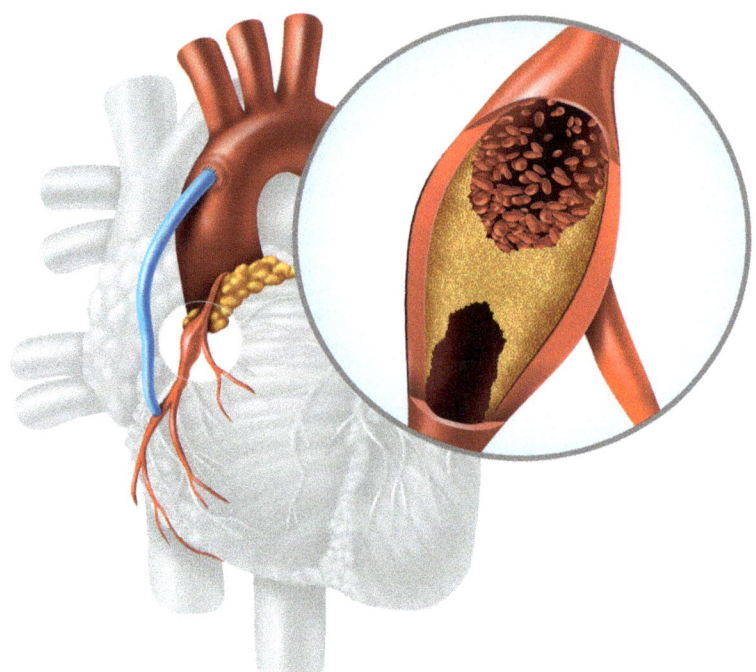

CABG Surgery

The coronary arteries deliver nutrients and oxygenated blood to the heart. As discussed earlier in the manuscript, atherosclerosis is a disease that can cause hardened plaque to build up in the coronary arteries. This plaque narrows the arteries over time.

This can limit the flow of blood to the heart and cause chest pain (angina). The plaque can also make blood clots more likely to form. These clots may completely block the blood flow through one of the arteries and cause a heart attack.

Off-pump CABG is one of the procedures that surgeons use to restore blood flow to the coronary arteries. The surgeon takes an artery or a vein from another place in the body. The surgeon then uses the vessel to "bypass" the blocked part of the vessel and restore normal blood flow to the heart. Your health-care provider may plan the surgery in advance, or you might need it in an emergency if a vessel suddenly becomes blocked.

Sometimes surgeons perform off-pump CABG with the traditional, standard surgical approach. In this type of CABG, the surgeon makes a large cut down the front of the chest through the breastbone (a sternotomy). Recently, some surgeons have started using smaller incisions to perform off-pump CABG. In this case, the surgeon makes a much smaller incision through the ribs to perform the surgery. This is a type of minimally invasive surgery. It is performed to reduce pain and recovery time.

Off-pump CABG may provide a slightly lower risk of complications than CABG performed with a heart-lung machine. Your particular risks will vary according to your particular medical conditions, your age, and other factors. In the off-pump technique, there may be a higher risk of needing another procedure to improve the heart's blood supply in the future. Be sure to talk with your health-care provider about any concerns that you have.

Most people who have off-pump CABG will have a successful outcome. However, there are some possible risks. These include the following:
- Infection
- Bleeding
- Irregular heart rhythms

- Blood clots leading to stroke or heart attack
- Complications from anesthesia
- Kidney failure

Certain factors increase the risk of complications. These include increased age and other medical conditions.

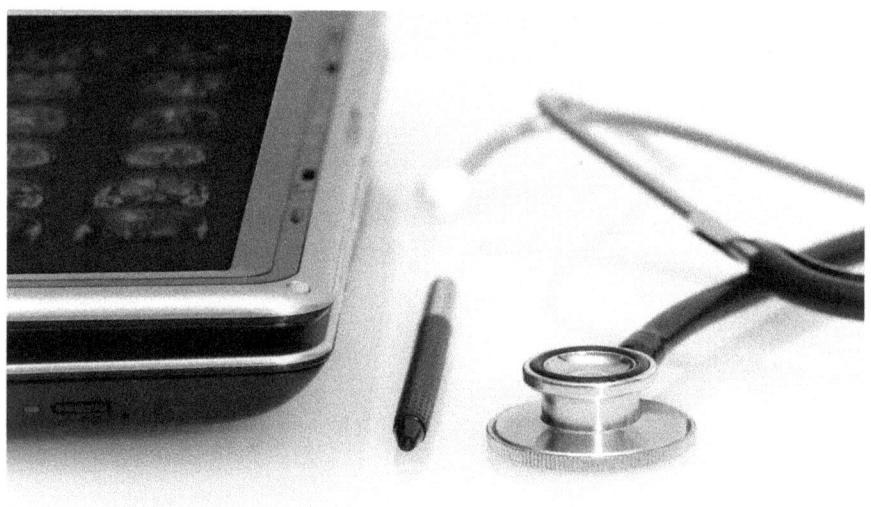

Stethoscope and Tablet PC

Talk with your health-care provider about how to get ready for your upcoming surgery. Remember the following:
- Avoid eating or drinking anything after midnight before your surgery.
- If you smoke, try to stop smoking before your operation.
- You may need to stop taking certain medicines, such as warfarin, before your surgery.
- Follow your health-care provider's instructions regarding medicine use before surgery.
- Check with your health-care provider about the details of your procedure.

In general, during your off-pump CABG, the following will happen:
- A health-care provider will give you anesthesia before the surgery starts. This will cause you to sleep deeply and painlessly during the operation. Afterward you won't remember the operation.
- The operation will take several hours.
- Your surgeon will make an incision to remove a vessel. Often this is a vessel taken from your chest wall or your leg.
- If you are having traditional off-pump CABG, your health-care provider will make an incision down the middle of your chest to separate your breastbone.
- If you are having a minimally invasive off-pump CABG, your surgeon may make a small incision down the middle of your chest and separate part of your breastbone. Sometimes surgeons use special instruments and a camera to do the surgery. In this approach, your health-care provider will make several small holes in your chest, between the ribs. Some surgeons use robot-controlled arms to perform the surgery.
- Your heart will keep beating during the surgery.
- Your surgeon will surgically attach the removed vessel to the aorta, the main blood vessel going out to the body. Your surgeon will attach the other end of the vessel to the blocked coronary artery to bypass the blockage. An artery inside the chest wall is typically used as the first bypass vessel of choice because it has been shown to stay open the longest.
- Once the bypass grafts are complete, a surgery team will wire your breastbone back together (if necessary).
- The surgery team will then sew or staple the incisions in your skin.

After your off-pump CABG, the following will happen:
- You might wake up a bit confused at first. You might wake up a couple of hours after the surgery or a little later.
- The surgery team will carefully monitor your vital signs, such as your heart rate. They may hook you up to several machines to assist in monitoring these continuously.
- You may have a tube in your throat to help you breathe. This may be uncomfortable, and you won't be able to talk. This will usually be removed within twenty-four hours.
- You may have a chest tube to drain excess fluid from your chest.
- You will feel some soreness, but you shouldn't feel severe pain. If you need it, you can ask for pain medicine.
- You should be able to sit in a chair and walk with help within a day or two.
- You may perform therapy to help remove fluids that collect in your lungs during surgery.
- You will probably be able to drink the day after surgery. You can have regular foods as soon as you can tolerate them.
- You will probably need to stay in the hospital around five days.

After you leave the hospital, the following will happen:
- Someone should drive you home from the hospital. For a while, you will also need some help at home.
- You will probably have your stitches or staples removed at a follow-up appointment in seven to ten days. Be sure to keep all follow-up appointments.
- You may still tire easily, but you will gradually start to recover your strength. It may be several weeks before you fully recover.

- Do not drive until your health-care provider says it is safe for you to do so.
- Avoid lifting anything heavy for several weeks.
- Follow all the instructions your health-care provider gives you for medicines, exercise, diet, and wound care.
- Your health-care provider may refer you to a cardiac rehab program to help in rebuilding your strength after surgery.

Carotid Endarterectomy

Carotid endarterectomy is a surgical procedure to remove a buildup of fatty deposits (plaque) that cause narrowing of the carotid artery. The carotid arteries are the main blood vessels that supply blood to the neck, face, and brain.

Carotid Angioplasty and Stenting

Carotid angioplasty and stenting are procedures that open clogged arteries to restore blood flow to the brain. They're often performed to treat or prevent strokes.

The carotid arteries are located on each side of your neck. These are the main arteries supplying blood to your brain. They can be clogged with fatty deposits (plaque) that slow or block blood flow to the brain—a condition known as carotid artery disease—which can lead to a stroke.

The procedure involves temporarily inserting and inflating a tiny balloon into the clogged artery to widen the area so that blood can flow freely to your brain.

Carotid angioplasty is often combined with another procedure called stenting. Stenting involves placing a small metal coil (stent) in the clogged artery. The stent helps prop the artery open and decreases the chance of it narrowing again. Carotid angioplasty and stenting may be used when traditional carotid surgery (carotid endarterectomy) isn't possible or it's too risky.

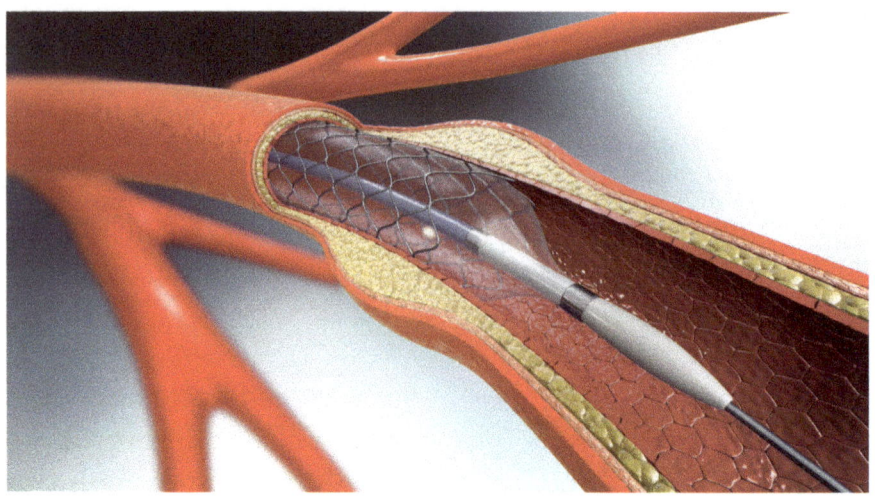

Arterial Stent Placement

The disruption in blood supply results in a lack of oxygen to the brain. This can cause sudden symptoms like those of a stroke. However, a TIA does not last as long as a stroke. The effects only last for a few minutes or hours and fully resolve within twenty-four hours.

A transient ischemic attack (TIA) is caused by a temporary state of reduced blood flow in a portion of the brain. This is most frequently caused by tiny blood clots that temporarily occlude a portion of the brain.

In an ischemic stroke, a blood clot blocks the blood supply to part of the brain. In a TIA, unlike a stroke, the blockage is brief, and there is no permanent damage.

Symptoms of a TIA are similar to those of a stroke, but they usually resolve quickly. If you notice any of the following symptoms, get medical attention right away:
- paralysis or weakness on one side of the body, usually in the face, arms, or legs
- difficulty speaking or understanding
- loss of balance or coordination, trouble walking

- trouble seeing out of one or both eyes
- confusion
- headache
- dizziness

Getting a medical evaluation within sixty minutes of the start of symptoms can help identify the cause of the TIA. This can help ensure that you get the right type of treatment, which may lower your risk of a future stroke.

According to research, up to 80 percent of strokes after a TIA are preventable, based on timely diagnosis and treatment.

In the event of an acute stroke, people who are able to get treatment within three hours of symptom onset experience better treatment outcomes with fewer long-term issues.

Anyone can have a stroke, but the following factors increase your risk:

- High blood pressure: high blood pressure is a leading cause of stroke and the most significant controllable risk factor.
- Diabetes: having either type 1 or type 2 diabetes doubles the risk of a stroke compared with someone without diabetes.
- High LDL cholesterol: having high levels of LDL cholesterol, also known as "bad" cholesterol, can cause cholesterol to build up in your arteries.
- Heart disease: some types of heart disease, especially atrial fibrillation (AFib), significantly increase the risk of stroke.
- Smoking: smoking damages your cardiovascular system and blood vessels, making it easier for blood vessels to rupture or for fatty material (plaque) to accumulate.
- Sex: men are more likely to have a stroke earlier in life than women. However, women tend to live longer than men, so they have a higher lifetime risk of stroke.

- Age: stroke can occur at any age, but your risk increases with age.
- Race and ethnicity: in the United States, stroke occurs more often in African American, American Indian, Alaska Native, and Hispanic adults than in White adults of the same age.

METABOLIC SYNDROME

Metabolic syndrome is a cluster of conditions that increases the risk of heart disease, stroke, and diabetes.

Metabolic syndrome includes high blood pressure, high blood sugar, too much body fat around the waist, and irregular cholesterol levels. The risk of metabolic syndrome increases with age. Hispanics also are at increased risk.

Most of the disorders associated with metabolic syndrome have no symptoms aside from a large waist circumference.

Weight loss, exercise, a healthy diet, and stopping smoking can help. Medicines also may be prescribed.

Causes of Metabolic Syndrome

Metabolic syndrome has several causes, and each affects the others. You can control some of these causes, such as your diet and physical activity levels. Other causes, such as your age and your genes, cannot be controlled.

The following lifestyle habits can raise your risk of metabolic syndrome:
- Being inactive
- Eating an unhealthy diet and large portion sizes
- Not getting enough good-quality sleep, which helps control how your body absorbs nutrients from the food you eat
- Smoking and drinking a lot of alcohol

A person's weight is another major cause of metabolic syndrome. Fat cells, especially in your abdomen, can raise your levels of chemicals called free fatty acids. Free fatty acids can raise your levels of other chemicals and hormones that affect the way your body controls your blood sugar levels. Your body may not respond well to insulin, which is a hormone that controls how much sugar your muscles and organs absorb from your blood. This is called insulin resistance.

Free fatty acids and insulin resistance can raise your "bad" LDL cholesterol and lower your "good" HDL cholesterol. Insulin resistance can also raise your blood pressure and blood triglyceride levels.

Also, cells from your immune system can cause your extra fat cells to make chemicals that increase inflammation in your body. This inflammation can cause plaque, a waxy substance, to build up inside your blood vessels. Plaque can break off and block your blood vessels. Inflammation itself also causes insulin resistance, high blood pressure, and heart and blood vessel diseases.

Prevention
The following steps can help you prevent metabolic syndrome:
- Maintain a healthy weight.
- Make heart-healthy lifestyle changes.
- Schedule routine health-care provider visits to keep track of your cholesterol, triglyceride, blood pressure, and blood sugar levels.
- Maintain a healthy BMI. Using the same cutoff in both sexes and in all age groups makes BMI simple and easy to use and interpret. However, a BMI of any level below 30 has a very high NPV to rule out metabolic syndrome. A BMI of 27 was found to be ideal for identification of metabolic syndrome in men and women.

Metabolic syndrome refers to the presence of a cluster of risk factors specific for cardiovascular disease. Metabolic syndrome greatly raises the risk of developing diabetes, heart disease, stroke, or all three.

According to the National Heart, Lung, and Blood Institute (NHLBI), the cluster of metabolic factors involved includes the following:

- Abdominal obesity. This means having a waist circumference of more than thirty-five inches for women and more than forty inches for men. An increased waist circumference is the form of obesity most strongly tied to metabolic syndrome.
- High blood pressure of 130/80 mm Hg (millimeters of mercury) or higher. Normal blood pressure is defined as less than 120 mm Hg for systolic pressure (the top number), and less than 80 mm Hg for diastolic pressure (the bottom number). High blood pressure is strongly tied to obesity. It is often found in people with insulin resistance.
- Impaired fasting blood glucose. This means a level equal to or greater than 100 mg/dL.
- High triglyceride levels of more than 150 mg/dL. Triglycerides are a type of fat in the blood.
- Low HDL (good) cholesterol. Less than 40 mg/dL for men and less than 50 mg/dL for women is considered low.

The NHLBI and American Heart Association (AHA) recommend a diagnosis of metabolic syndrome when a person has three or more of these factors.

Most people who have metabolic syndrome have insulin resistance. The body makes insulin to move glucose (sugar) into cells for use as energy. Obesity, commonly found in people with metabolic syndrome, makes it more difficult for cells in the body to respond to insulin. If the body can't make enough insulin to override the resistance, the blood sugar level increases, causing type 2 diabetes. Metabolic syndrome may be a start of the development of type 2 diabetes.

Because the population of the United States is aging, and because metabolic syndrome is more likely the older you are, the AHA has estimated that metabolic syndrome soon will become the main risk factor for cardiovascular disease, ahead of cigarette smoking. Experts also think that increasing rates of obesity are related to the increasing rates of metabolic syndrome.

Etiology of Metabolic Syndrome

Experts don't fully understand what causes metabolic syndrome. Several factors are interconnected. Obesity plus a sedentary lifestyle contributes to risk factors for metabolic syndrome. These include high cholesterol, insulin resistance, and high blood pressure. These risk factors may lead to cardiovascular disease and type 2 diabetes.

Because metabolic syndrome and insulin resistance are closely tied, many health-care providers believe that insulin resistance may be a cause of metabolic syndrome. But they have not found a direct link between the two conditions. Others believe that hormone changes caused by chronic stress lead to abdominal obesity, insulin resistance, and higher levels of blood lipids (triglycerides and cholesterol).

Other factors that may contribute to metabolic syndrome include genetic changes in a person's ability to break down fats (lipids) in the blood, older age, and problems in how body fat is distributed.

Risk Factors for Metabolic Syndrome

Knowing your risk factors for any disease can help guide you to take the appropriate actions. This includes changing behaviors and being monitored by your health-care provider for the disease.

Risk factors most closely tied to metabolic syndrome include the following:

- Age. You are more likely to have metabolic syndrome the older you are.
- Ethnicity. African Americans and Mexican Americans are more likely to get metabolic syndrome. African American women are about 60 percent more likely than African American men to have the syndrome.
- Body mass index (BMI) greater than 25. The BMI is a measure of body fat compared with height and weight.
- Personal or family history of diabetes. Women who have had diabetes during pregnancy (gestational diabetes) or people who have a family member with type 2 diabetes are at greater risk for metabolic syndrome.
- Smoking
- History of heavy drinking
- Stress
- Being past menopause
- High-fat diet
- Sedentary lifestyle

Symptoms of Metabolic Syndrome
Having high blood pressure, having high triglycerides, and being overweight or obese may be signs of metabolic syndrome. People with insulin resistance may have *acanthosis nigricans*. This is darkened skin areas on the back of the neck, in the armpits, and under the breasts. Some people do not have symptoms.

The symptoms of metabolic syndrome may look like those of other health conditions. See your health-care provider for a diagnosis.

Diagnosis of Metabolic Syndrome
Expert organizations have developed criteria to diagnose metabolic syndrome. Criteria include the following:
- Abdominal obesity

- BMI above 25
- High triglycerides
- Low HDL cholesterol
- High blood pressure or using medicine to lower blood pressure
- High fasting blood glucose
- Increased blood clotting. This means you have more plasma plasminogen activator and fibrinogen, which cause blood to clot.
- Insulin resistance. This means you have type 2 diabetes, impaired fasting glucose, or impaired glucose tolerance. The impaired glucose tolerance test measures the body's response to sugar.

Each organization has its own guidelines for using the above criteria to diagnose metabolic syndrome.

Treatment of Metabolic Syndrome

Your health-care provider will figure out the best treatment for you based on the following:
- How old you are
- Your overall health and past health
- How sick you are
- How well you can handle specific medicines, procedures, and therapies
- How long the condition is expected to last
- Your opinion or preference

Because metabolic syndrome increases the risk of developing more serious long-term (chronic) conditions, getting treatment is important. Without treatment, you may develop cardiovascular disease and type 2 diabetes. Other conditions that may develop as a result of metabolic syndrome include the following:
- Polycystic ovarian syndrome (PCOS)
- Fatty liver

- Cholesterol gallstones
- Asthma
- Sleep problems
- Some forms of cancer

Treatment usually involves lifestyle changes. This means losing weight, working with a dietitian to change your diet, and getting more exercise. Losing weight increases HDL ("good") cholesterol and lowers LDL ("bad") cholesterol and triglycerides. Losing weight can also reduce the risk for type 2 diabetes.

Losing even a modest amount of weight can lower blood pressure and increase sensitivity to insulin. It can also reduce the amount of fat around your middle. Diet, behavioral counseling, and exercise lower risk factors more than diet by itself.

Other lifestyle changes include quitting smoking and cutting back on the amount of alcohol you drink.

Diet

Changes in diet are important in treating metabolic syndrome. According to the AHA, treating insulin resistance is the key to changing other risk factors. In general, the best way to treat insulin resistance is by losing weight and getting more physical activity.

You can do this by doing the following: Include a variety of foods in your diet. Use healthy fats. Polyunsaturated and monounsaturated fats may help keep your heart healthy. These healthy fats are found in nuts, seeds, and some types of oils, such as olive, safflower, and canola.

Choose whole grains such as brown rice and whole-wheat bread instead of white rice and white bread. Whole-grain foods are rich in nutrients compared with more processed foods. Whole grains are higher in fiber, so the body absorbs them more slowly. They do not cause a rapid spike in insulin, which can trigger hunger and cravings. The 2015–2020 dietary guidelines from the USDA recommend that at least half your grains be whole grains.

Eat more fruits and vegetables. According to the 2015–2020 dietary guidelines, a person on a 2,000-calorie-per-day diet should eat 2.5 cups of vegetables and 2 cups of fruit a day. This amount will vary depending on how many calories you need. Be sure to choose a variety of fruits and vegetables. Different fruits and vegetables have different amounts and types of nutrients.

When eating out, take part of your restaurant meal home. When dining out or ordering takeout food, ask for a take-home box and avoid super-size selections when you order. Many restaurant portions are too large for one person, so consider sharing an entrée. Or order an appetizer instead of a main dish from the entrée menu.

Read food labels carefully. Pay close attention to the number of servings in the product and the serving size. If the label says a serving is 150 calories but the number of servings per container is three and you eat the entire container, you are getting 450 calories. Choose foods that are low in added sugar.

Exercise

Exercise helps people who are overweight or obese by helping to keep and add lean body mass, or muscle tissue, while losing fat. It also helps you lose weight faster than just following a healthy diet because muscle tissue burns calories faster.

Walking is a great exercise for just about anyone. Start slowly by walking thirty minutes daily for a few days a week. Gradually add more time so that you are walking for longer periods most days of the week.

Exercise lowers blood pressure and can help prevent type 2 diabetes. Exercise also helps you feel better emotionally, reduces appetite, improves sleep, improves flexibility, and lowers LDL cholesterol.

Talk with your health-care provider before starting any exercise program.

Medications
People who have metabolic syndrome or are at risk for it may need to take medications as treatment. This is especially true if diet and other lifestyle changes have not made a difference. Your doctor may prescribe medications to help lower blood pressure, improve insulin metabolism, lower LDL cholesterol and raise HDL cholesterol, increase weight loss, or some combination of these.

Weight-Loss Surgery
Weight-loss surgery (bariatric surgery) is an effective treatment for morbid obesity in people who have not been able to lose weight through diet, exercise, or medicine. It may also help people who are less obese but who have significant complications from their obesity.

Studies have shown that gastric bypass surgery helped lower blood pressure, cholesterol, and body weight at one year after the procedure.

Weight-loss surgery can be done in several ways, but all are either malabsorptive, restrictive, or a combination of the two. Malabsorptive procedures change the way the digestive system works. Restrictive procedures are those that greatly reduce the size of the stomach. The stomach then holds less food, but the digestive functions remain intact.

Prevention of Metabolic Syndrome
The best way to prevent metabolic syndrome is to maintain a healthy weight, eat a healthy diet, and be physically active. Your diet should have small amounts of salt, sugars, solid fats, and refined grains.

Living with Metabolic Syndrome
Metabolic syndrome is a lifelong condition that will require changes in your lifestyle. If you already have heart disease or

diabetes, follow your health-care provider's recommendations for managing these conditions.

Lifestyle changes involved in managing metabolic syndrome include the following:
- A healthy diet
- Physical activity and exercise
- Stopping smoking if you're a smoker or use other tobacco products
- Losing weight if you are overweight or obese

Key Points about Metabolic Syndrome

Below are some key points about metabolic syndrome:
- Metabolic syndrome is a condition that includes a cluster of risk factors specific for cardiovascular disease.
- The cluster of metabolic factors includes abdominal obesity, high blood pressure, impaired fasting glucose, high triglyceride levels, and low HDL cholesterol levels.
- Metabolic syndrome greatly raises the risk of developing diabetes, heart disease, stroke, or all three.
- Management and prevention of metabolic syndrome include maintaining a healthy weight, eating a healthy diet, eliminating the use of cigarettes or other tobacco products, and being physically active.

Next Steps

Here are some tips to help you get the most from a visit to your health-care provider:
- Know the reason for your visit and what you want to happen.
- Before your visit, write down questions you want answered.
- Bring someone with you to help you ask questions and remember what your provider tells you.

- At the visit, write down the name of a new diagnosis and any new medicines, treatments, or tests. Also write down any new instructions your provider gives you.
- Know why a new medicine or treatment is prescribed and how it will help you. Also know what the side effects are.
- Ask if your condition can be treated in other ways.
- Know why a test or procedure is recommended and what the results could mean.
- Know what to expect if you do not take the medicine or have the test or procedure.
- If you have a follow-up appointment, write down the date, time, and purpose for that visit.
- Know how you can contact your provider if you have questions.

The current medical approach is as follows: diabetes, cardiovascular disease, and cerebrovascular disease (stroke) are chronic, lifelong illnesses that progress and worsen with time. For example, once the diagnosis of diabetes is made, the standard initial treatment is metformin. Next there is increasing dosage of metformin to control the blood sugar. Then other medications may be added, such as saxagliptin, glyburide, glipizide, glimepiride, sitagliptin, rosiglitazone, pioglitazone, Ozempic, Wegovy, Moenjaro, Zepbound, and the like. Ultimately insulin is added to the regimen.

There is a minority of physicians and researchers who believe that these chronic diseases can be reversed and even prevented. They do not accept that these diseases are chronic and lifelong.

Here I will quote Dr. Azra Raza, author of *The First Cell*: "I predict a radical shift in all of health care in the coming decades. Early detection of neurologic, metabolic, cardiac, and oncologic diseases will naturally follow once we implement sensors designed to gauge disease-caused perturbation years ahead of their actual clinical appearances. This is how over the next few years, effective evidence-based preventive modalities will be developed, refined, and perfected."

I recommend the following books reflecting these views and providing hope for millions of people who suffer from chronic diseases.

1. *Life without Diabetes: Understanding and Reversing Type 2 Diabetes.* By Dr. Roy Taylor (a physician, diabetologist, and researcher).
2. *Outlive: The Science and Art of Longevity.* By Dr. Peter Attiya. *New York Times* bestseller.
3. *The Obesity Code* and *The Diabetes Code.* By Dr. Jason Fung.
4. *The First Cell: And the Human Costs of Pursuing Cancer to the Last.*

By Dr. Azra Raza.

Latest Update:

Some authorities have started to refer to this group of diseases as Adiposity based Chronic Diseases (ABCD). they believe that this terminology takes away the stigma and guilt. The patients will be more receptive of various modalities offered without the blame game.

GLOSSARY

Brain MRI: A brain MRI (magnetic resonance imaging) scan is a painless test that produces very clear images of the structures inside of your head—mainly, your brain.

A brain MRI can help doctors look for conditions such as bleeding, swelling, problems with the way the brain developed, tumors, infections, inflammation, damage from an injury or a stroke, or problems with the blood vessels. The MRI also can help doctors look for causes of headaches or seizures.

Carotid artery Doppler sonography: A carotid artery Doppler ultrasound is a diagnostic test used to check the circulation in the large arteries in the neck. This exam shows any blockage in the veins by a blood clot or "thrombus" formation. A carotid ultrasound is done to look for narrowed carotid arteries, which increase the risk of stroke.

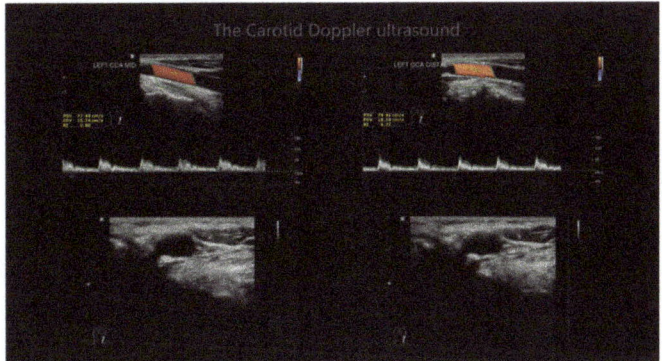

Carotid Artery Doppler Ultrasound

Coronary artery catheterization: During cardiac catheterization, a long, thin, flexible tube called a catheter is put into a blood vessel in your arm, groin or upper thigh, or neck. The catheter is then threaded through the blood vessels to your heart. It may be used to examine your heart valves or take samples of blood or heart tissue.

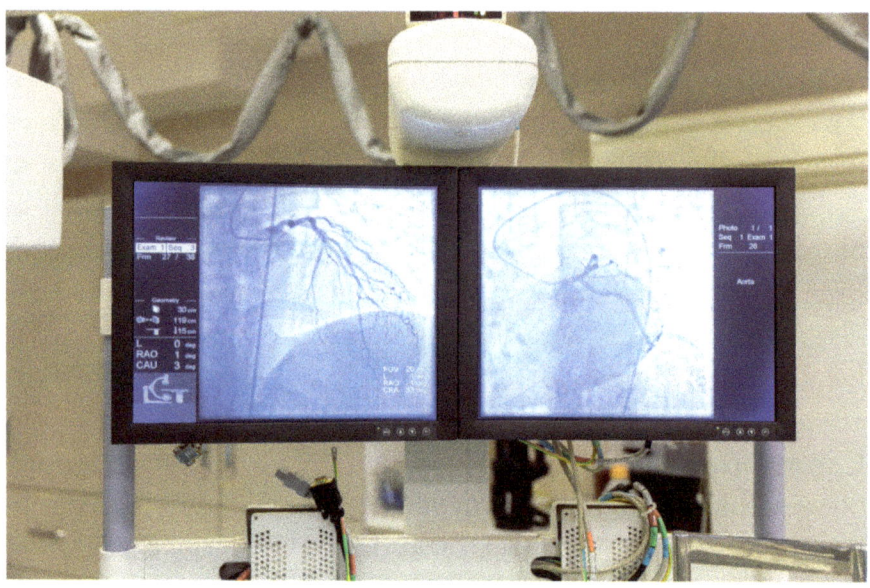

Coronary calcium scan: A coronary calcium scan is a special computerized tomography (CT) scan of the heart. It looks for calcium deposits in the heart arteries. This is typically most useful for people who don't yet have symptoms of heart disease but do have some risk factors. If your doctor is on the fence about how aggressively to treat you based on these risk factors, a CAC scan may help her or him determine the most appropriate treatment

CT carotid angiography with or without contrast injection: A carotid angiogram is a test to look at the large blood vessels in your neck that carry blood to your brain. These are called carotid arteries. The doctor puts a thin, flexible tube (catheter) into a blood vessel in your groin or arm. You may have this test to see if a carotid artery is narrowed.

A carotid CT angiogram uses a series of X-rays to diagnose vascular pathologies in the neck and brain and certain bone pathologies in the skull. In this case, a contrast agent is injected intravenously to highlight the area being examined.

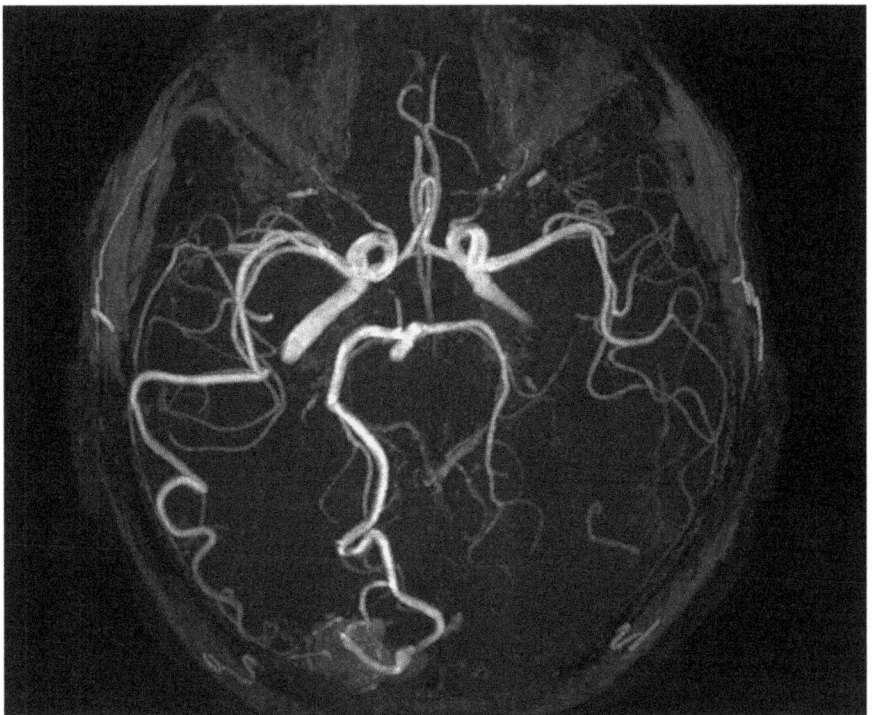

Cerebral Angiography from Flouroscopy

CT coronary angiography with or without contrast injection: A computerized tomography (CT) coronary angiogram is an imaging test that looks at the arteries that supply blood to the heart. A CT coronary angiogram uses a powerful X-ray machine to produce images of the heart and its blood vessels. The test is used to diagnose a variety of heart conditions.

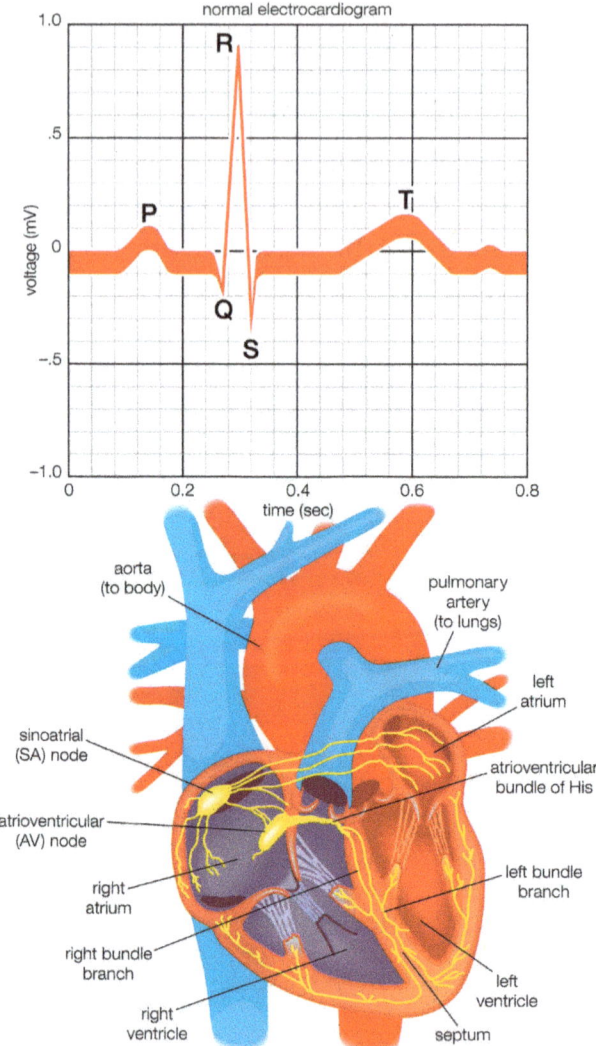

Electrocardiogram (ECG or EKG): An electrocardiogram is a simple, noninvasive test that records the electrical activity of the heart.

An electrocardiogram is a quick test to check the heartbeat. It records the electrical signals in the heart. Test results can help diagnose heart attacks and irregular heartbeats, called arrhythmias. ECG machines can be found in medical offices, hospitals, operating rooms, and ambulances.

Implantable loop recorder: An implantable loop recorder is a device that records the heartbeat continuously for up to three years. It's also called a cardiac event recorder. The device tells your care provider how the heart is beating while you do your daily activities.

The small device is placed just under the skin of the chest during a minor surgery.

Insertable cardiac monitor: A heart monitoring device.

Transesophageal echocardiography (TEE): A transesophageal echocardiogram uses echocardiography to assess the structure and function of the heart. During the procedure, a transducer (like a microphone) sends out ultrasonic sound waves.

MEDICAL TERMINOLOGY

Antiarrhythmic agents
Antihypertensive agents
Arteriosclerotic cardiovascular disease (ASCVD)
Cerebrovascular accident (CVA): stroke or transient ischemic attack (TIA)
Diabetes mellitus
Hypertension
Ischemic heart disease
Medical therapy for ASCVD
Myocardial infarction
Nitroglycerin—a coronary vasodilator
Statins

ACKNOWLEDGMENTS

Dearest Ammijan,

    I cannot thank AllahPak enough for blessing me with a mom like you. Your beauty, kindness, compassion, courage, love, and affection remain unmatched. You instilled in me a value system consisting of strong faith, independence of thought, and continual pursuit of knowledge to enlighten myself and achieve the best in life. Your guiding principles of honesty, fairness, humility, integrity, and forgiveness have proven helpful throughout my life and career. My dearest Ammijan, now that AllahPak has given me a second chance at life, I pledge to show you a better performance. Thanks for continuing to be my guardian angel from Jannah. Thanks, AllahPak, for giving me such parents. Given a choice, I would have chosen the same set. Hopefully I will not disappoint you when I see you again, inshallah.

> Umr bhar teri mohabbat meri khigmat ger rahi
> Mein teri Khidmat ke qabil jab hua tou chal basi
> Asman teri lahad per shabnam afshani karey
> Sabza e norasra eis ghar ki nigehbani karey.
>
> I was blessed to have such a dedicated and loving mother

Alas, I did not get an opportunity to reciprocate
May you rest in peace.

—Allama Iqbal

***

Dearest Abbajan,

    I am so thankful to AllahPak for blessing me with a father like you. Ammijan and you are the reason for my very existence and who I am. Thanks for instilling complete faith in AllahPak and intense love for the Holy Prophet and his progeny and for teaching me the value of knowledge and wisdom, hard work, honesty, integrity, equality, inclusion, and love. I am blessed to have seen all the value systems being practiced by you both. You taught me to help others, quietly keeping intact their self-respect. You taught me to appreciate poetry, literature, linguistics, reasoning, rationality, and always speaking the truth. I learned contemplation, reflection, and analytical thinking. I consider myself an experiment in progress you both started.

> Her aik se aashna houn laiken juda juda rasm o Raah meri
> Kisika Raqab, kissi ka Marqab, kissi ko ibrat ka taziana.

You taught me to be able to relate to everyone at their level.

—Allama Iqbal

ABOUT THE AUTHOR

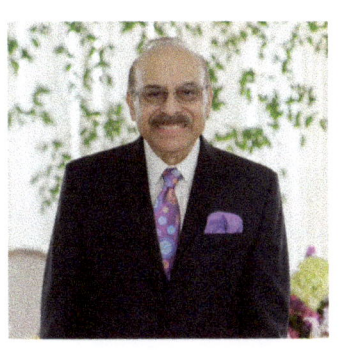

Dr. Jawad Hasnain, a distinguished anesthesiologist, pursued his medical studies at King Edward Medical University and later at the University of Maryland, specializing in Cardiovascular Anesthesiology. He achieved certification from the American Board of Anesthesiology and was accepted as a fellow of the American Colleges of Cardiology and Anesthesiology. He holds an MBA from the University of Maryland with twin majors in health informatics and international finance. With over 32 years as a faculty member at the University of Maryland he has made significant contributions to medical literature, particularly in Hemodynamic Monitoring, Thoracoscopy, Laparoscopy, and Transesophageal Echocardiography.

Now semi-retired, Dr. Hasnain continues his work as a locum anesthesiologist and is dedicated to combating obesity epidemic and metabolic syndrome. His book aims to personalize and humanize these health issues.

www.ingramcontent.com/pod-product-compliance
Lightning Source LLC
LaVergne TN
LVHW061631070526
838199LV00071B/6641